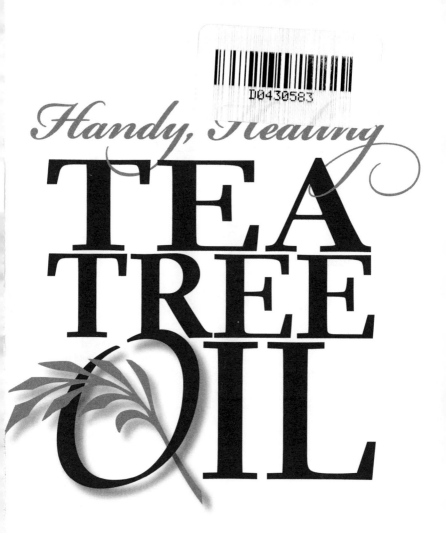

Handy, Healing

TEA TREE OIL

Joyce Johnson, ND

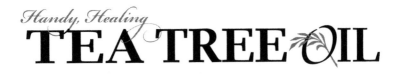

Mind Publishing

Our focus is education

FOR INFORMATION CONTACT
Mind Publishing Inc.
PO Box 57559, 1031 Brunette Avenue
Coquitlam, BC Canada V3K 1E0
Tel: 604-777-4330
Toll free: 1-877-477-4904
Fax: 1-866-367-5508
Email: info@mindpublishing.com
www.mindpublishing.com

ISBN 978-0-9782797-6-9
Printed in Canada

Contents

Legs and Feet 38

Summary 45

References 46

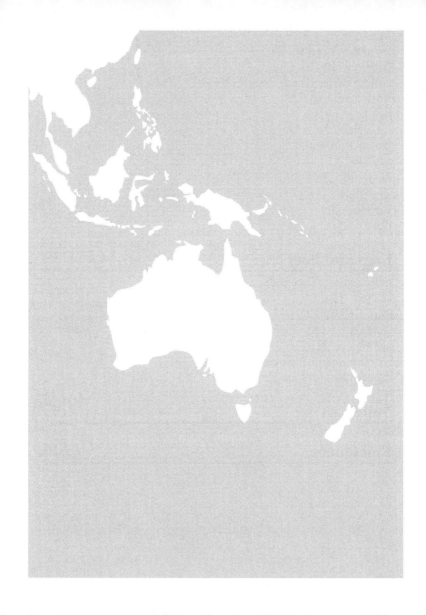

Introduction to Tea Tree Oil

Australia, one of the world's most popular travel destinations, has many claims to fame. On the natural health scene, one of the most valued exports from "down under" is an essential oil – commonly known as tea tree oil – from the *Melaleuca alternifolia* tree.

Once found only in Southeastern Australia, tea tree oil is fast becoming a global product. There are even plantations springing up in California. The trees grow to a height of approximately 20 feet, and while the whole tree is valued, only the leaves are used to produce the medicinal oil.

The Bundjalong aboriginal people of northern New South Wales Australia have known about the medicinal properties of this tree for centuries, but it wasn't until 1770 that the Western world started calling it the "tea tree" after Captain James Cook found its aromatic leaves an enjoyable substitute for real tea when he arrived in New South Wales. Gradually settlers, observing the locals, began to use the leaves, and the volatile oil obtained from them, in the treatment of cuts, abrasions, burns, insect bites, infections, and similar conditions.

The first official report of tea tree oil being used by a doctor was in the Medical Journal of Australia in 1930 where a Sydney surgeon wrote of its wound-healing and antiseptic properties.

During World War II, tea tree oil was added to machine "cutting" oils in munitions factories in Australia. This is said to have greatly reduced the number of infections on the hands of workers caused by abrasions from the metal filings and turnings (slivers).

The Many Uses of Tea Tree Oil

Tea tree essential oil is considered to be both antiseptic (able to destroy bacteria capable of causing infection) and antimicrobial (able to destroy or prevent the growth of microbes, microscopic living organisms that can include bacteria, fungi, parasites, and viruses). It is used medicinally in the treatment of many conditions, the most common being the prevention or treatment of acne, fungal infections, yeast infections, and a wide variety of skin conditions.

Tea tree oil works against bacteria and microbes in a similar way to disinfectants. It disrupts the cell membranes of destructive microorganisms and disables the proteins within them, basically "deactivating" them so they cannot multiply and cause health problems. The main active constituents in tea tree oil are chemical compounds terpinen-4-ol, alpha-terpineol, and linalool.

Using Tea Tree Oil
for Prevention and Treatment

Where can you use Tea Tree Oil? Everywhere!

This booklet is a handy guide that you can keep in your home, cottage, or office, or even your camper! You may be surprised at how many ways a small bottle of tea tree oil can be used. If you are unsure about what kind of tea tree oil to look for, I recommend a 100% pure undiluted tea tree oil from a trusted supplier. You should be able to find this useful essential oil wherever natural health products are sold.

To further assist you in overcoming any health challenges you identify while reading this book, I have included some additional nutritional supplement recommendations related to each condition or symptom. These are given in the interests of education and are not intended to prescribe, diagnose, or substitute for the advice of your health care practitioner.

In good health,
Joyce Johnson, ND

Head, Face, and Mouth

There are common health and cosmetic challenges that many people face (pardon the pun) related to hair, scalp, facial skin, lips, mouth, and teeth. In this section we look at some of the ways tea tree oil can help "at the top".

Acne (Acne vulgaris)

Acne is the most common skin problem in North America. One in four visitors to a dermatologist is there seeking help for this skin disorder, which can present as pimples, blackheads, and whiteheads, or as inflammatory acne with accompanying pustules and cysts. Inflammation occurs when the follicle (pore) wall is broken and white blood cells move in to fight bacteria. Acne breakouts frequently appear on the face, but can also be seen on the chest, back, and shoulders.

Acne generally begins at puberty because the production of androgens – hormones related to sexual development – causes a change in the size and activity of the sweat and sebaceous glands. Sebum is the semi-fluid oily mixture produced in your pores to keep the skin soft, flexible, and waterproof. Acne can be more than a cosmetic problem; it can cause emotional stress and have a profound impact on self-confidence. Tea tree oil is a naturally potent ally in the fight against acne.

Tea Tree Oil Remedy: Tea tree oil is a natural antiseptic and antibiotic. It has been shown to lower the level of bacteria and inflammation of acne as effectively as topical pharmaceutical medications, without negative side effects such as dry skin, redness, and peeling.

Dab a small amount of tea tree oil on blemishes three times per day. Alternatively, add 10 drops of tea tree oil to 60 mL (¼ cup) of warm water and wipe blemished areas morning and night with a clean cotton ball or pad.

Supporting Research: A clinical trial involving 124 patients with *Acne vulgaris* compared the use of tea tree oil to benzoyl peroxide over the course of three months. The tea tree oil product was significantly more effective at improving the acne and reducing the number of acne lesions. Tea tree oil was also better tolerated with fewer side effects such as dry skin, itchiness, and scaling skin.

Other Natural Remedies: In addition to using tea tree oil topically, acne may be improved by using these natural supplements, taken internally.

- Digestive enzymes
- Essential fatty acids
- Zinc
- Chromium
- Selenium
- Vitamin A
- Vitamin B complex
- Vitamin E
- Vitamin D
- Garlic

Canker Sores (*Aphthous stomatitis*)

Canker sores are a common condition. They are small white swellings in the mouth that can develop into ulcers. Outbreaks vary from a single sore, two or three times a year, to an uninterrupted succession of multiple sores. These small, shallow mouth ulcers are painful and can be quite annoying. They appear either singly or in clusters on the roof of the mouth, lips, gums, inner cheeks, tongue, and/or throat. The development of a canker sore may begin with a burning and tingling sensation. Canker sores typically heal without scarring within 1–3 weeks.

Tea Tree Oil Remedy: Tea tree oil is NOT to be swallowed or ingested. It can be dabbed onto canker sores with a clean cotton swab. Do not use full strength for children. Dilute 5–10 drops in 60 mL (¼ cup) of warm water and dab onto the canker sore.

Other Natural Remedies: In addition to using tea tree oil topically, canker sores may be prevented or relieved by using these natural supplements, taken internally.

- Acidophilus
- Vitamin B complex
- Zinc lozenges
- Deglycyrrhizinated licorice (DGL)
- L-lysine
- A good multivitamin
- Quercetin
- Vitamin C with bioflavonoids

Chapped Lips

Dry, cracked lips can be caused by a dry environment, excessive licking, or a reaction to irritants in cosmetics or skin treatments. Chapped lips can be painful and unattractive, and can interfere with basic day-to-day activities such as eating, talking, and kissing!

Tea Tree Oil Remedy: Add 5 drops of tea tree oil to your favourite lip balm or moisturizing cream. Apply to your lips as necessary, several times daily.

Other Natural Remedies:
- Increase water intake
- Essential fatty acids (e.g., fish oil, evening primrose oil)

Cold Sores (Herpes Simplex Virus 1)

Cold sores, also called "fever blisters", are the result of chronic, recurrent viral infections caused by the herpes simplex virus 1 (HSV-1), which is related to the virus that causes genital herpes. "Herpes" is from the Greek "to creep" and was used by Herodotus in 100 BC to describe fever blisters.

Cold sores typically appear on the lips, or on skin near the mouth, as single or multiple small bumps filled with fluid, within 3–10 days after exposure to the herpes virus. They can last up to, or longer than, three weeks. Cold sores can spread and grow, and are painful, itchy, and irritating. Unfortunately, the virus remains in the body permanently, which is why some people are prone to frequent outbreaks. It is estimated that 80% of the population have been exposed to HSV-1 and have antibodies against it. Strengthening immunity is important to preventing outbreaks.

Tea Tree Oil Remedy: Tea tree oil can speed the healing of cold sores. Apply a few drops using a cotton swab as soon as you feel the tenderness and itching that usually precede a cold sore. If the cold sore is already "in full bloom" apply a few drops of tea tree oil to the infected area twice a day.

Supporting Research: A randomized, placebo-controlled study involving 20 patients with cold sores (herpes labialis) investigated the effectiveness of a tea tree oil product and reported that it had benefits over the placebo. An in vitro study has also demonstrated the activity of tea tree oil against the herpes simplex viruses 1 and 2.

Other Natural Remedies: Cold sores and other viral infections are most likely to occur when the immune system is weak or compromised. Strengthen your immunity and, in addition to using tea tree oil topically, use these natural supplements, taken internally, for long-term health benefits.

- L-lysine
- Acidophilus
- Zinc
- Vitamin C with bioflavonoids
- Vitamin B complex
- Garlic
- Vitamin A

Common Cold (Rhinovirus)

Affecting the upper respiratory tract, the common cold is caused by a virus. Contrary to popular belief, cold weather and being exposed to drafts or temperature changes do NOT cause colds. Cold viruses survive better in colder temperatures, so they tend to thrive in the fall and winter months. Cold sufferers experience symptoms such as head congestion, runny nose, sore throat, sneezing, coughing, headache, and watery eyes. The majority of colds resolve on their own within 7–10 days, but occasionally they can lead to more serious illnesses involving the lungs (bronchitis, pneumonia), the ears (middle ear infections), and the sinuses.

Tea Tree Oil Remedy: Add 5–10 drops of tea tree oil to 960 mL (4 cups) of very hot water in a pot. Make a "steamer" by draping a towel over your head and over the pot. Inhale the steam to clear the breathing passages. At night add 10 drops of tea tree oil to your vaporizer. You can also rub a drop on under your nose and on each temple. Eucalyptus oil is another soothing oil for steam inhalation.

Other Natural Remedies: In addition to using tea tree oil topically, help your body prevent or shorten the duration of colds by using these natural supplements, taken internally.

- Echinacea
- Selenium
- Zinc/zinc lozenges
- Garlic
- A good multivitamin/ multimineral
- Vitamin E
- Vitamin A
- Vitamin C with bioflavonoids
- Maitake extract

Dandruff

Dandruff is a common condition of the scalp that occurs when skin cells renew themselves and the dead skin is shed or sloughed off, resulting in annoying, often itchy, white flakes. Dandruff is more common with oily, rather than dry, skin. Everyone produces and sheds skin cells at different rates. New research shows that severe cases of dandruff may be caused by an overgrowth of a yeast called *Pityrosporum ovale* that naturally resides on the skin.

Tea Tree Oil Remedy: Add 20 drops of tea tree oil to your shampoo bottle and mix; use daily or alternate with another shampoo. Or use 3 drops of tea tree oil mixed with your shampoo in your hand. Rubbing a few drops of tea tree oil directly onto the scalp may help unblock the hair follicles.

Supporting Research: A 4-week trial involving 126 patients with dandruff reported that a product containing 5% tea tree oil was more effective than the placebo and was well tolerated.

Other Natural Remedies: Preventing or treating dandruff and other skin/scalp conditions can be easier if you consume adequate nutrients. The following supplements can improve scalp and hair health.

- Essential fatty acids
- Selenium
- Vitamin B6
- Vitamin E
- Vitamin A
- Kelp
- Vitamin B complex
- Vitamin B12
- Zinc
- Vitamin C with bioflavonoids

Dental Care

The mouth is a breeding ground for bacteria. It is warm, moist, and full of nooks and crannies where bacteria can hide, producing bad breath and promoting gum disease and tooth decay. Sore throats, canker sores, and mouth ulcers are all too common.

Tea tree oil is NOT to be swallowed, so any oral use must be approached with care. Although some natural health care practitioners recommend adding tea tree oil to your toothbrush or mouthwash, or rinsing with it, I suggest using a commercial tea tree oil toothpaste or mouthwash rather than risking ingesting too much of this potent oil.

Other Natural Remedies: Brushing the teeth regularly and flossing can do a lot for mouth health, as can regular rinsing with hot water and salt, or a natural mouthwash. Nutritional supplements can include immune builders such as vitamin C and L-lysine, and echinacea and zinc lozenges can improve a sore throat.

Ear Infections/Earaches

Approximately 75% of all children suffer from ear infections by the age of three. There are two types of ear infections that doctors encounter in their practices, otitis externa and otitis media. Otitis media, also known as swimmer's ear, affects the outer ear and can include symptoms such as a slight fever, discharge, and pain. Otitis media, a middle ear infection, is very common in infants and children, and is an infection located behind the eardrum. This is where the small bones of the ear are located. If a bacteria or virus invades this region, inflammation and fluid buildup, creating a sensation of pressure. Symptoms include earache, high fever, sharp, throbbing pain, and a feeling of fullness in the ear.

Tea Tree Oil Remedy: For otitis externa, mix 5 drops of tea tree oil in 60 mL (¼ cup) of warm olive oil. Drop a small amount gently into the ear, tilting the head to one side for a minute. Use a small cotton ball or swab, gently, to absorb the oil. Repeat until improved.

Other Natural Remedies: Prevention is important and a strong immune system is your best protection against infections. The following supplements support immunity and fight infections:

- Zinc
- Vitamin B complex
- Echinacea
- Vitamin C with bioflavonoids
- Vitamin E

Gum Disease (*Gingivitis*)

Gingivitis is a condition in the periodontal disease (pyorrhea) group. It involves inflammation of the gums and is the early stage of periodontal disease. The main cause of gingivitis is poor hygiene characterized by plaque – deposits of bacteria, mucus, and food particles stuck to the teeth.

Tea Tree Oil Remedy: As mentioned above, tea tree oil is NOT to be swallowed. Use a natural, commercial tea tree oil toothpaste or mouthwash rather than risking ingesting too much of this potent oil.

Other Natural Remedies: Brushing the teeth regularly and flossing can do a lot for mouth health, as can regular rinsing with hot water and salt, or a natural mouthwash. The following nutritional supplements can also improve gum health:

- Coenzyme Q10
- Calcium and magnesium
- Vitamin B complex
- Vitamin A
- Lactobacillus rinse
- Vitamin C with bioflavonoids
- Zinc
- Grape seed extract
- Vitamin E

Head Lice/Scabies

Scabies is an infestation of the skin by parasitic itch mites, which burrow under the skin and lay eggs, causing a persistent, itchy rash. Lice, on the other hand, live on an individual or in their clothing. Scabies mites are transmitted from person to person, usually from prolonged contact, whereas lice are transmitted from person to person and also from bedding and clothing.

Scabies is characterized by intense itching, skin burrows, and occasionally secondary infections, with the most severe itching occurring at bedtime. The lesions and burrows are seen in the finger webs, wrists, beltline, groin, areola in females, and lower buttocks.

Lice may produce tiny black specks in undergarments and nits (lice eggs) may be seen at the base of hair shafts. Mild excoriations (abraded skin) may be visible from scratching.

Tea Tree Oil Remedy: For head lice, add 5 drops of tea tree oil to 30 mL (1 oz) of shampoo. Massage into the hair, leave on for 10 minutes, rinse; repeat once a day until nits and lice are gone. This shampoo can also be used on other areas affected by lice or scabies. Tea tree oil may be applied directly, twice a day, to an area affected by scabies, but it could cause irritation in people with sensitive skin. Consult a health care practitioner if an improvement is not seen within 10 days.

Supporting Research: In test tube studies, topical application of tea tree oil was very effective against head lice with 93% of lice and 83% of nits destroyed.

Other Natural Remedies:
- Vitamin A
- Kelp
- Evening primrose oil
  (for scabies)
- Garlic
- Zinc

Oral Thrush

Thrush is a fungal infection of the mouth characterized by creamy-white patches which form on the tongue and mucous membranes. Scraping the patches off can cause bleeding. Oral thrush is most commonly seen in infants, or individuals with compromised immune systems.

Tea Tree Oil Remedy: I do not recommend gargling with tea tree oil, or other oral uses, unless you use a natural, commercially prepared rinse or mouthwash. You may get relief by "steaming" over a pot of hot water with 5–10 drops of tea tree oil added.

Other Natural Remedies:
- Acidophilus
- Vitamin B complex
- Vitamin E
- Essential fatty acids
- Vitamin C with bioflavonoids
- Garlic
- Echinacea
- Zinc
- Vitamin A

Sinusitis

Sinusitis is an inflammation of the nasal sinuses. The most common cause of sinusitis is a viral upper respiratory infection, although bacteria, fungi, and allergic reactions may also be responsible. Any factor that creates swelling of the nasal tissues, resulting in obstruction and the lack of proper drainage of the area, will often lead to a sinus infection. Chronic sinusitis is most common in people with allergies, and dental infections account for 25% of chronic maxillary sinusitis. Swimming and diving, as well as injury to the area (especially a broken nose affecting the frontal sinuses) are other precipitating factors.

Tea Tree Oil Remedy: Add 5–10 drops of tea tree oil to a pot of heated water. Drape a towel over your head. Lean over the pot and inhale gently. At night, add 10 drops to a vaporizer.

Other Natural Remedies: Sinusitis may respond to the following dietary supplements due to their antibacterial, anti-inflammatory, or antioxidant actions.

- Acidophilus
- Flaxseed oil
- Quercetin
- Zinc
- Vitamin A
- A good multivitamin/ multimineral
- Bee pollen
- Coenzyme Q10
- Bromelain
- Vitamin B complex
- Vitamin C with bioflavonoids

Throat, Chest, and Body

Some of the tips in Section 1 will also apply to these parts of the body, but there are other ways tea tree oil can improve your mobility, flexibility, breathing, and immunity.

Arthritis (Osteoarthritis and Rheumatoid Arthritis)

Arthritis means inflammation of one or more joints. Osteoarthritis is the degeneration and loss of cartilage in the joints, with accompanying stiffness and pain. Osteoarthritis is the most common form of arthritis and can affect all the joints, but has special affinity for the weight-bearing joints (knees, hips, and spine). It is seen in both men and women. It usually occurs in men before 45 years of age, and in women after 45–55 years of age. Osteoarthritis is very common and may have hereditary causes, but factors such as poor diet, trauma, and repetitive forceful stress to a joint seem to precipitate arthritic conditions.

Rheumatoid arthritis is a chronic form of arthritis that can lead to destruction of the bone and cartilage, resulting in characteristic deformities. It can appear in many forms: from a mild short-lasting illness that causes little damage, to a severe, progressive disease causing significant joint destruction. Rheumatoid arthritis occurs in about 1% of the population, about three times more often in women than in men. RA usually occurs between the ages of 35–50 and has a genetic association.

Tea Tree Oil Remedy: For joint swelling and pain due to arthritis, add 10 drops of tea tree oil to 60 mL (2 oz) of jojoba or grapeseed oil and massage affected areas 2–3 times daily. Tea tree oil appears to be able to penetrate the joint and desensitize irritated nerve endings.

Other Natural Remedies:

Osteoarthritis:

- Glucosamine sulfate
- MSM
- S-adenosyl-L-methionine (SAMe)
- Essential fatty acids (e.g., omega-3s from fish or flaxseed oils)
- Bromelain
- Chondroitin sulfate
- Celadrin
- A good multivitamin/ multimineral
- Turmeric

Rheumatoid Arthritis:

- Quercetin
- Vitamin E
- Bromelain
- Essential fatty acids (e.g., omega-6 from evening primrose oil, and omega-3s from fish and flaxseed oils)
- Celadrin
- Betaine HCL
- Selenium
- Vitamin C
- A good multivitamin/ multimineral

Bladder Infection (Cystitis)

Bladder infections are acute inflammations/infections of the urinary bladder. They are very common and occur in females 10 times more often than in males, except during infancy when both sexes are equally affected. Symptoms include painful urination or a feeling that you have to urinate but cannot.

More severe bladder infections can cause back pain and fever. Cranberry and blueberry extracts are excellent oral supplements for urinary tract infections.

Tea Tree Oil Remedy: It is important to keep the urethra and genital area clean to prevent infections or shorten their duration. Add 3 drops of tea tree oil to 120 mL (½ cup) of purified or distilled water and wash genital area thoroughly. Put 10 drops of tea tree oil into hot bath water for a soothing soak.

Other Natural Remedies:

- Cranberry or blueberry concentrated extracts
- Acidophilus and bifidus probiotics
- B complex
- Garlic
- Uva ursi herbal extract (*Arctostaphylos uva ursi*)
- A good multivitamin/ multimineral
- Vitamin C with bioflavonoids
- Zinc

Bronchitis

Bronchitis is an infection of the trachea (windpipe) and bronchioles ("branches") that usually follows an upper respiratory infection like a cold or cough. Bronchitis is most common in the winter. Other factors that contribute to developing bronchitis include air pollution, chronic sinusitis, and irritating fumes (acute irritative bronchitis) such as ammonia, smoke, and chlorine.

Tea Tree Oil Remedy: Add 3 drops of tea tree oil to a warm, damp cloth and apply to chest, or add 10 drops of tea tree oil to a hot bath and soak.

Other Natural Remedies:
- Vitamin C
- Echinacea
- Vitamin B complex
- Coenzyme Q10
- Greens powder
- A good multivitamin/ multimineral
- Vitamin A
- Zinc
- Quercetin
- MSM
- N-acetylcysteine (NAC)

Bruises

A bruise is formed when tissues below the skin are injured due to physical trauma. The skin remains intact, but the capillaries carrying blood below the surface are broken and blood is able to drain into surrounding tissue. People who do not consume enough fresh, uncooked foods to provide the body with needed nutrients are more likely to bruise easily.

Tea Tree Oil Remedy: Apply ice if swelling occurs. Mix 5 drops of tea tree oil into an arnica or comfrey salve. Apply daily as needed.

Other Natural Remedies:

- Iron (if anemic)
- Alfalfa
- Vitamin B complex
- A good multivitamin/ multimineral
- Coenzyme Q10
- Vitamin E
- Vitamin D
- Vitamin C with bioflavonoids

Burns

The skin is the body's largest organ, which makes a serious burn one of the most traumatic injuries the body can sustain. First-degree burns involve the surface of the skin. They can cause mild pain, redness, dry skin, and swelling. No blisters form and healing usually occurs without scarring in 2–3 days. An example would be a typical sunburn.

Second-degree burns involve deeper layers of the skin, including the upper level of the dermis. Skin functions are lost, blisters form, pain and swelling occur, and healing can take 7–10 days with possible scarring.

Third-degree burns include destruction of both the epidermis and dermis. Skin functions are lost, and there is no pain in the immediate area of the burn due to the destruction of nerve endings, although there may be extreme pain in surrounding tissue. Regeneration of the skin following a third-degree burn is slow and may require skin grafts, leaving an obvious scar.

Tea Tree Oil Remedy: Tea tree oil can help speed healing of a minor, first-degree burn. Immediately wash the area with ice water, and apply a few drops of tea tree oil to the burned area. Repeat 3–4 times daily. For a healing salve, mix 20 drops of tea tree oil with 90 mL (3 oz) of raw unpasteurized honey and 2.5 mL (½ tsp) triple strength grapefruit seed extract.

Other Natural Remedies:

Topically:
- Calendula
- Aloe vera gel

Orally:
- Potassium
- Vitamin A
- Vitamin B complex
- Vitamin C with bioflavonoids
- Vitamin E
- Zinc
- Essential fatty acids
- Coenzyme Q10
- Calcium and magnesium with vitamin D

Coughs

Congestion in the lungs, from viral infections or irritation, can result in coughing, with or without excess mucous and phlegm.

Tea Tree Oil Remedy: Add 6–8 drops of tea tree oil to 960–1440 mL (4–6 cups) of warm water. Drape a towel over your head, lean over the warm water, and gently inhale the vapours for 10 minutes. At night you can add 10 drops of tea tree oil to the water in a vaporizer and let it steam for 5–10 minutes.

Other Natural Remedies:
- Natural cough syrups with horehound, wild cherry, mullein, eucalyptus, and honey.
- Zinc lozenges

Cuts and Wounds

Cuts, scrapes, and puncture wounds are common occurrences, especially in children. Any serious injury should be seen by a health care professional, but most minor cuts and wounds can be treated at home. Any injury that involves broken skin should be kept clean to avoid infection.

Tea Tree Oil Remedy: Tea tree oil should not be applied directly to open cuts or wounds, but a diluted mixture (10 drops in 240 mL [1 cup] of warm water) may be applied as an antiseptic wash, or onto a cloth bandage if the cut or wound is stitched or closed.

Other Natural Remedies:
- Calendula
- Vitamin E oil

Dermatitis/Eczema

Dermatitis is the general name given to any inflammation of the skin. Often the terms dermatitis and eczema are used interchangeably. Eczema can be caused by a number of things such as stress, fatigue, and nutrient deficiency, all of which play a role in allowing environmental or internal irritants to cause various skin conditions.

Tea Tree Oil Remedy: Tea tree oil is a natural antiseptic and antibiotic. It can lower the level of bacteria on the skin without negative side effects such as dry skin, redness, and peeling. However, depending on the severity of the condition, you may want to test a small patch of skin before using tea tree oil broadly, to determine sensitivity.

Dab a small amount of tea tree oil onto an affected area. If no irritation occurs, repeat on other areas. You can also add 10 drops of tea tree oil to 60 mL (¼ cup) of warm water and wash affected areas morning and night with a clean, 100% cotton ball or pad, then pat until dry.

Other Natural Remedies:
- Betaine HCL´
- Kelp
- Vitamin E
- Acidophilus
- Vitamin D
- Quercetin
- MSM
- Vitamin C with bioflavonoids
- Zinc
- Vitamin A
- Vitamin B complex
- Selenium

- Essential fatty acids
  (e.g., omega-6 from evening
  primrose oil, and omega-3s
  from fish and flaxseed oils)
- Vitamin B complex

- Zinc oxide (topically) with
  vitamin E

Hemorrhoids

Hemorrhoids are swollen (varicose) veins around the anus
and in the rectum that may protrude from the anus. If the
hemorrhoids are located inside the anal canal, they are called
internal hemorrhoids. If located at the anal opening, they are
called external hemorrhoids.

Factors that increase your risk of hemorrhoid formation include:
- Heredity
- Standing for long periods
  of time
- A sedentary lifestyle
- Straining during bowel
  movements or chronic
  constipation

- Pregnancy
- Benign prostatic hypertrophy
  (enlarged prostate)
- Sitting on hard, cold surfaces
- Liver stagnancy or liver
  disease (cirrhosis)

Tea Tree Oil Remedy: Apply a mixture of tea tree oil (about
5 drops) and a natural oil like olive or almond oil to the affected
area twice daily.

Other Natural Remedies:

- Vitamin B complex
- Ground flaxseed
- Calcium and magnesium
- Vitamin C with bioflavonoids
- Flaxseed oil
- Psyllium seed powder
- Vitamin E

Genital Herpes (Herpes Simplex Virus 2)

Genital herpes is the most common sexually transmitted disease. On average, one out of every five people over the age of 12 has it, although more than half never develop serious symptoms. Systemic symptoms include fever, muscle pain, general malaise, and headaches. Genital complaints include pain (can be severe), itching, and vaginal and urethral discharge. In women, most initial infections involve the cervix and urethra. People who already have cold sores caused by HSV-1 may have a less intense primary attack of genital herpes. Recurrences of genital herpes are common, usually within 1–4 months of the first outbreak; the average number of recurrences is 4–7 per year.

Tea Tree Oil Remedy: Mix 2 drops of tea tree oil with the contents of 1 capsule of natural source vitamin E and apply to herpes lesions twice daily. Discontinue use if irritation occurs. You can also add 10 drops of tea tree oil to bath water or to a "sitz" bath (a seated bath where only the hips and buttocks are submerged).

Supporting Research: An in vitro study has demonstrated activity of tea tree oil against the HSV-1 and -2.

Other Natural Remedies: The following supplements can help improve immunity and reduce the frequency or severity of HSV-1 and -2 attacks.

Orally:

- L-lysine
- Vitamin A
- Zinc
- Essential fatty acids
- Vitamin E
- Vitamin C with bioflavonoids
- Vitamin B complex
- Acidophilus
- Garlic

Topically:

- Licorice root (Glycyrrhiza)
- Topical vitamin E and zinc

Hives (Urticaria)

Hives is a skin condition characterized by sudden outbreaks of red, itchy welts. Hives are relatively common, with about 15–20% of the population experiencing them. Although seen in people of all ages, hives seem to be more prevalent among young adults (from post-adolescence until 30 years of age). The reaction is basically an allergic response. Hives usually resolve within a few hours to a couple of days, but in rare cases they become chronic and may last for six weeks or more.

Tea Tree Oil Remedy: Add 4 drops of tea tree oil to 60 mL (2 oz) of witch hazel. Massage affected area.

Other Natural Remedies:

- Acidophilus
- Vitamin B complex
- Quercetin
- Essential fatty acids
  (e.g., omega-6 from evening
  primrose oil, and omega-3s
  from fish and flaxseed oils)
- Vitamin D
- Garlic
- Vitamin C with bioflavonoids
- Vitamin E
- A good multivitamin/
  multimineral

Jock Itch

Fungal infections of the skin commonly occur in places that are moist and where one skin surface is in contact with another. Jock itch is a fungal infection of the skin in the groin area.

Tea Tree Oil Remedy: Apply several times per day to the affected area, either full strength or diluted with distilled water or cold-pressed vegetable oil.

Other Natural Remedies:

- Acidophilus
- Vitamin B complex
- Vitamin E
- Essential fatty acids
- Garlic
- Vitamin C with bioflavonoids
- Zinc
- Vitamin A

Laryngitis

Laryngitis is an inflammation of the larynx. Most laryngitis is caused by microorganisms, both viral and bacterial (especially streptococcus). It can also occur concurrently with other infections such as urinary tract infections and lung infections. Other causes include voice overuse, allergic reactions, and inhaling irritating substances (e.g., smoking).

Tea Tree Oil Remedy: I do not recommend gargling with tea tree oil, except if you use a natural, commercially prepared rinse or mouthwash. You may get relief by "steaming" over a pot of hot water with 5–10 drops of tea tree oil added.

Other Natural Remedies:
- Vitamin C   - Vitamin A
- Zinc, zinc lozenges

Muscle Pain

Overexertion or sudden straining can cause muscles to become inflamed and tender. Some of the healing actions of tea tree oil are apparently able to penetrate the skin and ease sore muscles.

Tea Tree Oil Remedy: Mix 5 drops of tea tree oil with 30 mL (1 oz) of grapeseed oil. Massage well. You can also add 10 drops to bath water and soak.

Other Natural Remedies:
- Creatine
- Calcium and magnesium
- L-glutamine

Psoriasis

Psoriasis is one of the most common chronic skin diseases. Most people experience the onset before the age of 20. Psoriasis appears as patches of skin on the legs, knees, arms, elbows, scalp, ears, and back that are red to brown in colour and covered with silvery-white scales. There seems to be a genetic tendency, as 30% of people with psoriasis have a family history that includes psoriasis. The exact cause is unknown.

Tea Tree Oil Remedy: Tea tree oil is a natural antiseptic and antibiotic. It can lower the level of bacteria on the skin without negative side effects such as dry skin, redness, and peeling. However, depending on the severity of the psoriasis, you may want to test a small patch of skin before using tea tree oil broadly, to determine sensitivity.

Dab a small amount of tea tree oil on an affected area. If no irritation occurs, repeat on other areas. You can also add 10 drops of tea tree oil to 60 mL (¼ cup) of warm water and wash affected areas morning and night with a clean 100% cotton ball or pad, then pat until dry.

Other Natural Remedies:

- Zinc
- Chromium
- Vitamin D
- MSM
- Selenium
- A good multivitamin/
  multimineral
- Vitamin A
- Vitamin E
- Vitamin B complex
- Vitamin C with bioflavonoids
- Milk thistle
- Essential fatty acids
  (e.g., omega-6 from evening
  primrose oil, and omega-3s
  from fish and flaxseed oils)

Ringworm

Ringworm, also known as a tinea infection, is not a worm, but a fungal infection that occurs on the skin or scalp. It is characterized by the appearance of small red spots that increase in size to approximately ¼ inch in diameter. Ringworm can be extremely itchy.

Tea Tree Oil Remedy: Apply tea tree oil to affected areas, full strength, twice daily. Stop use if irritation occurs.

Other Natural Remedies:

- Acidophilus
- Vitamin B complex
- Vitamin E
- Essential fatty acids
- Garlic
- Vitamin C with bioflavonoids
- Zinc
- Vitamin A

Sore Throat

One of the most common health complaints, sore throats can vary from a raw, burning, scratching feeling to a sense of fullness and discomfort when swallowing. Viral infections are the most common culprits when it comes to sore throats, which often go hand-in-hand with the common cold. However, sore throats can also be caused by substances that irritate the back of the throat.

Tea Tree Oil Remedy: I do not recommend gargling with tea tree oil, except if you use a natural, commercially prepared rinse or mouthwash. You may get relief by "steaming" over a pot of hot water with 5–10 drops of tea tree oil added. A hot water and salt gargle is also effective.

Other Natural Remedies:
- Acidophilus
- Garlic
- Vitamin E
- Zinc lozenges
- A good multivitamin/ multimineral
- Bee propolis
- Maitake extract
- Vitamin C with bioflavonoids
- Echinacea
- Vitamin A

Vaginitis

Vaginitis is an infection of the vaginal tract that causes inflammation of the vaginal lining. Although vaginitis can be caused by a sexually transmitted infectious micro-organism, it is more typically due to a disturbance in the delicate ecology of the vagina that allows organisms normally found in a healthy vagina to overgrow and produce an infection.

Tea Tree Oil Remedy: Apply a few drops of the oil on a tampon, or mix with water and use as a douche. Topical tea tree oil cream can also be used.

Supporting Research: In 2003 the World Health Organization stated that clinical data supported the use of tea tree oil for vaginitis and cervicitis. A study found that intravaginal application of tampons soaked in a diluted tea tree oil solution successfully healed vaginitis and cervicitis in 130 patients with a *Trichomonas vaginalis* infection. Vaginal "suppositories" containing 0.2 g tea tree essential oil, inserted nightly, eradicated symptoms in women with *Candida albicans* vaginitis after 30 days in 86% of women, with a full 75% free of infection.

Other Natural Remedies:

Orally:
- Acidophilus
- Garlic
- Vitamin B complex
- Selenium
- Vitamin D
- A good multivitamin/ multimineral

- Echinacea
- Essential fatty acids
- Vitamin E
- Vitamin A
- Vitamin E
- Zinc

Topically:
- Aloe vera

- Calendula and vitamin A suppositories

Warts

Warts are small growths caused by human papilloma viruses (HPV). Although warts may occur at any age, they are most common in older children and are rarely seen in the elderly. Warts can be found anywhere in the body, but are most commonly found on the hands, fingers, elbows, forearms, knees, face, and skin around the nails.

Tea Tree Oil Remedy: Apply full strength tea tree oil to the wart. It may take several weeks for the wart to dissolve

Other Natural Remedies:

- Vitamin B complex
- Vitamin E
- MSM
- A good multivitamin/
  multimineral

- Vitamin A
- Vitamin C with bioflavonoids
- Zinc

Legs and Feet

They carry us around all day and are often ignored when it comes to tender loving care, but our legs and feet need love too! Tea tree oil's popularity doesn't stop at athlete's foot, although that is one of the most common uses of this potent natural ally.

Athlete's Foot *(Tinea pedis)*

Athlete's foot is a tinea infection, one that thrives in an environment that is warm and moist. The fungus lives off the dead skin cells and calluses of the feet, especially between the toes. It is very common in gyms, swimming pools, and locker rooms. Symptoms can range from simple peeling of the skin, to deep cracking with severe itching and inflammation.

Tea Tree Oil Remedy: Soak feet in a foot bath with 20 drops of tea tree oil for 15 minutes, three times daily (or as often as possible). Dry feet off thoroughly and apply tea tree oil, full strength, to affected areas.

Supporting Research: In a double-blind, randomized trial of 158 patients with athlete's foot, the effectiveness of two strengths of tea tree oil (25% and 50%) were compared. After applying the tea tree oil twice daily for four weeks, the authors concluded that both strengths were effective. The 25% tea tree oil preparation had fewer complications and was more highly recommended by the authors of the study.

Another double-blind, randomized trial treated 104 patients with athlete's foot using either a 10% tea tree oil cream, a 1% tolnaftate cream, or a placebo cream. This study showed that the tolnaftate caused the greatest reduction in the fungal infection, however the tea tree oil cream was just as effective at reducing symptoms.

Other Natural Remedies:

- Acidophilus
- Vitamin B complex
- Zinc
- Vitamin A
- Garlic
- Vitamin C with bioflavonoids
- Essential fatty acids
- Vitamin E

Blisters

A blister is rather like a friction burn on the skin, and it can easily become infected if the skin breaks. Keep the area clean and cover with a bandage if necessary.

Tea Tree Oil Remedy: Apply full-strength tea tree oil to the affected area.

Corns and Calluses

Corns and calluses are an overgrowth of skin tissue (hyperkeratosis) that eventually thickens and hardens. Calluses occur most commonly on areas that incur a lot of friction, such as the soles of the feet and the hands. Corns are cone-shaped overgrowths and most often form between the toes. These growths can cause inflammation and pain.

Tea Tree Oil Remedy: Add 3 drops of tea tree oil to 5 mL (1 tsp) grapeseed, apricot, olive, almond, or avocado oil. Massage well into the corn or callus, or soak the feet in a mixture of 10 drops tea tree oil and 15 mL (½ oz) grapeseed, apricot, olive, almond, or avocado oil for 5 minutes, twice daily. Once the corn or callus has become soft, remove with tweezers and apply a few drops of tea tree oil, then cover with a bandage.

Other Natural Remedies:
- Topical vitamin E oil

Gout

Gout is a common form of arthritis which typically first appears in the first joint of the big toe. It is a protein metabolism disorder which leads to an increased concentration of uric acid. In gout, uric acid crystals (monosodium urate) are deposited in joints, tendons, kidneys, and other tissues, causing considerable inflammation and damage. Kidney involvement may lead to kidney failure. Gout occurs more commonly in men.

Tea Tree Oil Remedy: For joint swelling caused by gout, mix 5 drops of tea tree oil with 60 mL (2 oz) of jojoba or grapeseed oil and massage into the affected area 2–3 times daily.

Other Natural Remedies:
- Chondroitin
- Vitamin E
- Bromelain
- Quercetin
- Kelp or alfalfa
- Omega-3
- Folic acid
- Devil's claw
- Vitamin B complex
- Vitamin C with bioflavonoids

- Grape seed extract
- Calcium and magnesium
- A good multivitamin/
  multimineral
- MSM

- Zinc
- Glucosamine
- Celadrin (oral and topical
  forms are available)

Leg Ulcers

When the legs experience poor circulation, blood flow is restricted, the skin tissue can erode and ulcers form. Due to the poor circulation, healing leg ulcers can be quite slow. Leg ulcers tend to occur in individuals with poor circulation, such as diabetics.

Tea Tree Oil Remedy: Apply 8 drops of tea tree oil to 720 mL (3 cups) of warm water or add 5 drops of tea tree oil to 30 mL (1 oz) of grapeseed oil. Shake well and massage into affected area.

Other Natural Remedies:
- Coenzyme Q10
- Grape seed extract
- Vitamin E
- Zinc
- A good multivitamin/
  multimineral

- Garlic
- Vitamin C with bioflavonoids
- Flaxseed oil
- Echinacea
- Vitamin B complex

Nail Infections
(Paronychia and Onychomycosis)

Paronychia is an infection that develops along the edge of the fingernail or toenail. Fungal infections under the nails can cause the nail to rise off the nail bed, swelling of the nail bed and discolouration of the nail. Onychomycosis is a fungal infection of the nail that results in thickening, roughness, and splitting of the nails. It can lead to a complete destruction of the nail. Both these infections may improve with the use of tea tree oil.

Tea Tree Oil Remedy: Apply 2–3 drops of tea tree oil directly to the nail and surrounding tissue. Repeat every morning and night, or more frequently when possible. These infections can be persistent, so you must be as well.

Supporting Research: A randomized, controlled trial of 117 patients suffering from onychomycosis compared the effectiveness of tea tree oil to a topical medication (1% clotrimazole cream) over a 6-month period. Improvements in both groups were comparable, as was the cost of the treatments. A second randomized, double-blind, placebo-controlled trial involving 60 patients with onychomycosis compared a combination cream (containing 5% tea tree oil and 2% butenafine hydrochloride) to a placebo. At the end of the 16-week trial, 80% of those who used the tea tree oil preparation were cured, compared to no cures at all in the placebo group.

Other Natural Remedies:

- Acidophilus
- Vitamin B complex
- Vitamin E
- Essential fatty acids
- Silica
- Garlic
- Vitamin C with bioflavonoids
- Zinc
- Vitamin A
- Calcium and magnesium
  with vitamin D

Plantar Warts

Plantar warts are usually found on the soles of the feet and the underside of the toes. They are characterized by white raised growths that resemble calluses and interrupt the natural "footprint." They can be tender to the touch and may bleed if scraped or trimmed.

Tea Tree Oil Remedy: Apply full strength tea tree oil to the affected area 2–3 times daily.

Other Natural Remedies:

- Vitamin B complex
- Vitamin E
- MSM
- A good multivitamin/
  multimineral
- Vitamin A
- Vitamin C with bioflavonoids
- Zinc

Topical Remedy: You can also try the "tape occlusion" technique (also called the "Red-Green approach"). Apply duct tape over the wart for approximately two months, changing periodically.

Summary

More than any other single "herb", the essential oil of the tea tree has gathered a following of dedicated users who continue to find new ways to use this simple product to enhance their lives or help prevent illness and infections. I haven't touched on the ways this unique oil can be added to household products for cleaning and disinfecting – but that doesn't mean you can't look into those as well.

There are many different concentrations of tea tree oils and lotions available. There are tea tree oil shampoos and conditioners. There is everything from tea tree oil lip balm to tea tree oil toothpaste. Enjoy trying a variety of tea tree oil products for your home and family.

One last word of warning: Do NOT use tea tree oil on your pets. It could be harmful to them and is not advised. Veterinarians trained in holistic medicine have products appropriate for your pet's good health.

Joyce Johnson, ND

References

Altman P. Australian tea tree oil. *Aust. J. Pharm.* 1988; 69:276-78.

Balch PA. *Prescription for Nutritional Healing.* 4th ed. New York, NY: Penguin Books Limited; 2006.

Bassett IB, Pannowitz DL, Barnetson RS. A comparative study of tea-tree oil versus benzoylperoxide in the treatment of acne. *Med J Aust.* 1990; 153(8):455-458.

Belaiche P. Letter to the Editor. *Phytotherapy Res.* 1988; 2:157.

Blackwell AL. Tea tree oil and anaerobic (bacterial) vaginosis. *Lancet.* 1991; 337.8736:300.

Brown D. Topical tea tree oil for onychomycosis. *Quarterly Review of Natural Medicine.* 1995; Spring:11.

Boon H, Smith M. *The Complete Natural Medicine Guide to the 50 Most Common Medicinal Herbs.* Toronto: The Institute of Naturopathic Medicine and Research (The Canadian College of Naturopathic Medicine); 2004.

Braun L, Cohen M. *Herbs and Natural Supplements – An evidence-based guide.* Elsevier Health Sciences; 2004.

Brown D. Tea tree oil for athlete's foot. *Quarterly Review of Natural Medicine.* 1993; Winter:15.

Buck DS, Nidorf DM, Addino JG. Comparison of two topical preparations for the treatment of onychomycosis: *Melaleuca alternifolia* (tea tree) oil and clotrimazole. *J Fam Pract.* 1994; 38: 601-605.

Carson CF, Ashton L, Dry L, et al. *Melaleuca alternifolia* (tea tree) oil gel (6%) for the treatment of recurrent herpes labialis. *J Antimicrob Chemother.* 2001; 48(3):450-51.

Concha JM, Moore LS, Holloway WJ. 1998 William J. Stickel Bronze Award. Antifungal activity of *Melaleuca alternifolia* (tea tree) oil against various pathogenic organisms. *J Am Podiatr Med Assoc.* 1998; 88.10:489-92.

Cox SD et al. The mode of antimicrobial action of the essential oil of *Melaleuca alternifolia* (tea tree oil). *J Appl Microbiol.* 2000; 88.1:170-75.

Gustafson JE et al. Effects of tea tree oil on *Escherichia coli. Lett Appl Microbiol.* 1998; 26.3:194-98.

Hammer KA, Carson CF & Riley TV. Susceptibility of transient and commensal skin flora to the essential oil of *Melaleuca alternifolia* (tea tree oil). *Am J Infect Control.* 1996; 24.3:186-89.

Hammer KA, Carson CF & Riley TV. In vitro activity of essential oils, in particular *Melaleuca alternifolia* (tea tree) oil and tea tree oil products, against Candida spp. *J Antimicrob Chemother.* 1998; 42.5:591-95.

Hammer KA, Carson CF & Riley TV. In vitro activities of ketoconazole, econazole, miconazole, and *Melaleuca alternifolia* (tea tree) oil against Malassezia species. *Antimicrobial Agents and Chemotherapy.* (2000); 44:467-469.

Jacobs MR, Hornfeldt CS. Melaleuca oil poisoning. *J Toxicol Clin Toxicol.* 1994; 32.4:461-64.

Prepubertal Gynecomastia Linked to Lavender and Tea Tree Oils. *N Engl J Med.* 2007; 356:479-485.

Leung AY, Foster S. *Encyclopedia of Common Natural Ingredients used in Food, Drugs, and Cosmetics.* 2nd ed. Toronto, ON/New York, NY: John Wiley and Sons Inc; 1996.

Murray M. *The healing power of herbs.* 1995, Prima Health, USA.

Pizzorno L, Pizzorno J, Murray M. *Natural Medicine Instructions for Patients.* Elsevier Health Sciences; 2002.

Satchell AC, Saurajen A, Bell C, et al. Treatment of interdigital tinea pedis with 25% and 50% tea tree oil solution: a randomized, placebo-controlled, blinded study. *Australasian J Dermatol.* 2002; 43(3):175-178.

Satchell AC, Saurajen A, Bell C, et al. Treatment of dandruff with 5% tea tree oil shampoo. *J Am Acad Dermatol.* 2002; 47(6):852-855.

Schnitzler P, Schon K, Reichling J. Antiviral activity of Australian tea tree oil and eucalyptus oil against herpes simplex virus in cell culture. *Pharmazie.* 2001; 56.4:343-47.

Syed TA, Qureshi ZA, Ali SM, et al. Treatment of toenail onychomycosis with 2% butenafine and 5% *Melaleuca alternifolia* (tea tree) oil in cream. *Trop Med Int Health.* 1999; 4(4):284-287.

Tisserand R, Balacs T. *Essential Oil Safety: A Guide for Health Care Professionals.* London: Churchill Livingstone; 1995.

Tong MM, Altman PM, Barnetson RSt.-C. Tea tree oil in the treatment of Tinea pedis. *Australian J Dermatology.* 1992; 33:145-149.

Tyler VE, Robbers JE. Tyler's Herbs of Choice. *The Therapeutic Use of Phytomedicinals.* Binghampton, NY: The Haworth Herbal Press; 2000.

Tyler VE. *Tyler's Honest Herbal.* 4th ed. Binghampton, NY: The Haworth Herbal Press; 2000.

Veal L. The potential effectiveness of essential oils as a treatment for headlice, *Pediculus humanus capitis. Complement Ther Nurs Midwifery.* 1996; 2.4:97-101.

Walton SF, et al. Acaricidal Activity of *Melaleuca alternifolia* (Tea Tree) Oil. In Vitro Sensitivity of *Sarcoptes scabiei var hominis* to Terpinen-4-ol. *Arch Dermatol.* 2004; 140:563-566.

Williams L, Home VA. A comparative study of some essential oils for potential use in topical applications for the treatment of the yeast *Candida albicans. Australian Journal of Medical Herbalism.* 1995; 7(3):57-62.